TUBERCULOSIS

THINGS YOU SHOULD KNOW
(QUESTIONS AND ANSWERS)

By Rumi Michael Leigh

Introduction

I would like to thank and congratulate you for purchasing this book, " *Tuberculosis, things you should know (questions and answers)*" series.

This book will help you understand, revise and have a good general knowledge and keywords of Tuberculosis and how it affects the lives of people who suffer from this disease.

Thanks again for purchasing this book, I hope you enjoy it!

Chapter 1

1) What is the abbreviation of tuberculosis ?

- TB is the abbreviation of tuberculosis.

2) How does tuberculosis stay in the air ?

- Tuberculosis stays in the air as water droplets.

3) How long can the water droplets of tuberculosis stay in the air ?

- The water droplets of tuberculosis can stay several hours in the air.

4) What are some systemic symptoms of tuberculosis ?

- Some systemic symptoms of tuberculosis are fatigue, weight loss, sweating, fever, etc.

5) What part of the lungs does tuberculosis usually affect ?

- Tuberculosis usually affects the upper part of the lungs.

6) Why does tuberculosis affect the upper part of the lungs ?

- Tuberculosis usually affects the upper part of the lungs because the upper part of the lungs contains more oxygen.

7) Where does tuberculosis travel in order to reach other organs ?

- Tuberculosis travels by the lymph nodes and the blood.

8) What is an active tuberculosis infection ?

- An active tuberculosis infection is when there is multiplication of bacteria.

9) Where does active tuberculosis start ?

- Active tuberculosis starts in the lungs.

Chapter 2

1) What are the bacteria that cause tuberculosis ?

- The bacteria that cause tuberculosis is the mycobacterium.

2) What are aerobes ?

- Aerobes are microorganisms that need oxygen to survive.

3) What do mycobacterium need to survive ?

- Mycobacterium need oxygen to survive.

4) Do people who are infected with tuberculosis always have symptoms ?

- No, people who are infected with tuberculosis do not always have symptoms.

5) Why are people who are infected with tuberculosis not always aware of this disease ?

- People who are infected with tuberculosis are not always aware of this disease because the infection can remain latent for a long time.

6) What can cause a tuberculosis infection to leave its latent form to an active form ?

- A disease such as HIV/AIDS can cause a tuberculosis infection to leave its latent form to an active form. This happens when the immune system is compromised.

7) Should latent tuberculosis infection be treated ?

- Yes, latent tuberculosis infection should be treated.

8) Why should latent tuberculosis infection be treated ?

- Latent tuberculosis infection should be treated in order to prevent tuberculosis disease.

9) What is a primary infection of tuberculosis ?

- A primary infection of tuberculosis is tuberculosis in its latent phase.

10) Is latent TB contagious ?

- No, latent tuberculosis is not contagious.

Chapter 3

1) What is systemic miliary tuberculosis ?

- Systemic miliary tuberculosis is when tuberculosis spreads to other tissues of the body.

2) How can systemic miliary tuberculosis affect the kidneys ?

- Systemic miliary tuberculosis can cause sterile pyuria.

3) What is sterile pyuria ?

- Sterile pyuria is the presence of white blood cells in the urine without a known presence of urinary tract infection.

4) How can systemic miliary tuberculosis affect the brain ?

- Systemic miliary tuberculosis can cause meningitis.

5) What is meningitis ?

- Meningitis is an infection that causes inflammation of the meninges.

6) What are meninges ?

- Meninges are the membranes around the brain and the spinal cord.

7) Why are patients with tuberculosis meningitis and tuberculosis pericarditis given steroids ?

- Patients with tuberculosis meningitis and tuberculosis pericarditis are given steroids in order to reduce inflammation.

8) How can systemic miliary tuberculosis affect the adrenal glands ?

- Systemic miliary tuberculosis can cause Addison's disease.

9) What is Addison's disease ?

- Addison's disease is when the adrenal glands don't produce enough hormones.

10) How can systemic miliary tuberculosis affect the liver ?

- Systemic miliary tuberculosis can cause hepatitis.

Chapter 4

1) What is another name for white blood cells ?

- Another name for white blood cells is leucocytes.

2) What is hemoptysis ?

- Hemoptysis is the coughing of blood.

3) What is a sputum ?

- A sputum is a thick mucus mixed with saliva coughed from the lungs.

4) What is another name for the mucus of a sputum ?

- Another name for the mucus of a sputum is phlegm.

5) What is hyperuricemia ?

- Hyperuricemia is a high level of uric acid in the blood.

6) What is optic neuritis ?

- Optic neuritis is the inflammation of the optic nerve.

7) What is mycetoma ?

- Mycetoma is a chronic inflammatory disease caused by certain bacteria or fungi on the skin and subcutaneous tissue.

8) What is bronchiectasis ?

- Bronchiectasis is the abnormal widening and scarring of the airways.

9) What are alveoli ?

- Alveoli are tiny air sacs of the lungs.

10) What is the function of alveoli ?

- Alveoli allow gas exchange.

Chapter 5

1) What is pulmonary tuberculosis ?

- Pulmonary tuberculosis is a serious bacterial infection of the lungs.

2) What is extrapulmonary tuberculosis ?

- Extrapulmonary tuberculosis is tuberculosis elsewhere in the body apart from the lungs.

3) What is tuberculosis osteomyelitis ?

- Tuberculosis osteomyelitis is tuberculosis infection of the bone.

4) What is another name for tuberculosis osteomyelitis ?

- Tuberculosis osteomyelitis is also called Pott's disease.

5) Where does tuberculosis osteomyelitis usually occur ?

- Tuberculosis osteomyelitis usually occurs in the vertebrae.

6) What is arthritis ?

- Arthritis is an inflammation of the joints.

7) What is Gout ?

- Gout is a form of arthritis that causes severe pain due to a high level of uric acid in the blood.

8) What is a joint ?

- A joint is a place where two or more bones meet.

9) What is bacteriostatic ?

- Bacteriostatic means stopping the reproducing process of bacteria.

10) What is bactericide ?

- Bactericide means the killing of bacteria.

Chapter 6

1) What are the common tests for detecting tuberculosis ?

- The common tests for detecting tuberculosis are chest X-ray, sputum examination, and culture.

2) What is the best test to diagnose tuberculosis ?

- The best test to diagnose tuberculosis is the culture test.

3) What is the disadvantage of the culture test for the diagnosis of tuberculosis ?

- The disadvantage of the culture test for the diagnosis of tuberculosis is that it takes a lot of time. It could take weeks.

4) Is a chest X-ray for a person with latent tuberculosis normal ?

- Yes, a person with latent tuberculosis has a normal chest X-ray.

5) Is a chest X-ray for a person with active tuberculosis normal ?

- No, a person with active tuberculosis has an abnormal chest X-ray.

6) How is a sputum sample collected ?

- A sputum sample can be collected by a patient's cough or by bronchoscopy.

7) What is the best time to take a sputum sample from a patient ?

- The best time to take a sputum sample from a patient is before a patient has breakfast.

8) Is the sputum test for a person with latent tuberculosis positive or negative ?

- The sputum test for a person with latent tuberculosis is negative.

9) Is the sputum culture positive or negative for a person with latent tuberculosis ?

- The sputum culture is positive for a person with latent tuberculosis.

10) Is the sputum culture positive or negative for a person with active tuberculosis ?

- The sputum culture is positive for a person with active tuberculosis.

11) Is the tuberculin skin test positive or negative for a person with latent tuberculosis ?

- The tuberculin skin test is positive for a person with latent tuberculosis.

12) Is the tuberculin skin test positive or negative for a person with active tuberculosis ?

- The tuberculin skin test is positive for a person with active tuberculosis.

Chapter 7

1) What is the abbreviation PPD ?

- Purified Protein Derivative.

2) What is PPD ?

- PPD is a skin test for tuberculosis.

3) Where is PPD injected ?

- PPD is injected in the forearm.

4) What is another name for the PPD test ?

- The PPD test is also called the Mantoux test.

5) What kind of needle is used to inject PPD ?

- A tuberculin needle is used to inject PPD.

6) Does a positive result of PPD always signify an active tuberculosis ?

- No, a positive result of PPD does not always signify an active tuberculosis.

7) What are the most common treatments of active tuberculosis ?

- The most common treatments of active tuberculosis are Pyrazinamide, Rifampin, Ethambutol, and Isoniazid.

8) What happens when a patient skips his tuberculosis medications ?

- Skipping tuberculosis medication can make the bacteria more resistant to the medications.

9) What are some of the signs of a patient on Rifampin ?

- A patient on Rifampin can have red secretions such as tears and urine.

10) What is the function of Rifampin ?

- Rifampin kills bacteria.

Chapter 8

1) How does Isoniazid work ?

- Isoniazid kills bacteria.

2) Why does Isoniazid cause symptoms such as depression, fatigue, etc. ?

- Isoniazid causes symptoms such as depression, fatigue, etc. because it decreases the level of vitamin B6 in the body.

3) How does Pyrazinamide work ?

- Pyrazinamide kills bacteria.

4) What is a common treatment of active tuberculosis that can cause hyperuricemia ?

- Pyrazinamide is a common treatment of active tuberculosis that can cause hyperuricemia.

5) What is a common treatment of active tuberculosis that can cause optic neuritis ?

- Ethambutol is a common treatment of active tuberculosis that can cause optic neuritis.

6) How does Ethambutol work ?

- Ethambutol kills bacteria.

7) How does Streptomycin work ?

- Streptomycin kills bacteria.

8) What is an important side effect of Streptomycin?

- Streptomycin can cause hearing loss.

Chapter 9

1) What are the immune cells that protect the alveoli when there is the presence of bacteria ?

- Macrophages are the immune cells that protect the alveoli when there is the presence of bacteria.

2) What does "phage" mean ?

- Phage means to eat.

3) Do macrophages always destroy bacteria in a tuberculosis infection ?

- No, macrophages sometimes do not succeed in destroying all the bacterial infections.

4) What is a granuloma ?

- A granuloma is a granulation tissue formed due to an inflammation or an infection.

5) What is another name for granuloma ?

- Tuberculoma is another name for granuloma.

6) What is a Gohn focus ?

- A Gohn focus is a visible and large granuloma.

7) What is a Gohn complex ?

- A Gohn complex is a combination of an infected granuloma and a regional lymph node.

8) What are ototoxic drugs ?

- Ototoxic drugs are drugs that are toxic to the ears.

9) How long is the treatment for active tuberculosis?

- The treatment for active tuberculosis can take from 6 months to a year.

Chapter 10

1) What is the abbreviation IGRA ?

- Interferon Gamma Release Assay.

2) Name the two types of Interferon Gamma Release Assay.

- The two types of Interferon Gamma Release Assay are T-Spot and Quantiferon TB Gold (QFT) test.

3) What is the advantage of the Interferon Gamma Release Assay over the Purified Protein Derivative test ?

- The advantage of the Interferon Gamma Release Assay test over the Purified Protein Derivative test is that the results are immediate.

4) Does the Interferon Gamma Release Assay test show if the patient has a latent or an active tuberculosis ?

- No, the interferon Gamma Release Assay test does not show if the patient has a latent or active tuberculosis.

5) Does the Purified Protein Derivative test show if the patient has latent or active tuberculosis ?

- No, the Purified Protein Derivative test does not show if the patient has a latent or an active tuberculosis.

6) In what kind of environment are patients with active tuberculosis treated ?

- Patients with active tuberculosis are treated in isolation.

7) Why are patients with active tuberculosis treated in isolation ?

- Patients with active tuberculosis are treated in isolation because they are highly contagious.

8) When can a patient come out of the isolation state ?

- A patient can come out of the isolation state when they have been on regular medication for at least three weeks and there are signs of improvement on their sputum culture, and there is improvement in the signs and symptoms of their disease.

9) What is the abbreviation dot ?

- Directly Observed Therapy.

10) What is the use of the directly observed therapy ?

- The directly observed therapy is used to control the patient's intake of their medications in order to ensure compliance.

Conclusion

Thank you again for purchasing this book. I hope it has helped you in your journey to understanding Tuberculosis and how it affects the people around you who suffer from it.

Thank you.